TESTS
AND
MEASUREMENTS
FOR
BEHAVIORAL
OPTOMETRISTS

Harold A. Solan, O.D., M.A.
Professor, State College of Optometry
State University of New York

Irwin B. Suchoff, O.D.
Professor, State College of Optometry
State University of New York

OPTOMETRIC EXTENSION PROGRAM
CURRICULUM II

Copyright © 1991 Optometric Extension Program Foundation, Inc.

Printed in the United States of America

Published by the Optometric Extension Program Foundation, Inc.
2912 South Daimler Street
Santa Ana, CA 92705-5811

Managing Editor: Sally Marshall Corngold
Illustrator: Marcia Castaneda

Library of Congress Cataloging-in-Publication Data Pending

ISBN 0-943599-21-0

TABLE OF CONTENTS

Proceeds from the sale of this text are donated

to

the Homer H. Hendrickson Memorial Fund

at the request of the authors

Harold A. Solan, O.D., M.A.

and

Irwin B. Suchoff, O.D.

PROLOGUE

The monograph began as a journal article. However, it soon became apparent that because of the nature of Tests and Measurements, our purpose, to make a complicated area of knowledge comprehensible and useful for optometric clinicians, could not be met in a single, or even several journal articles. This option would have mandated that we write a relatively cursory overview of all aspects of the subject, in which case only those individuals with a prior knowledge of Tests and Measurements would benefit. We then explored the option of writing a textbook. The downside risk here was that it would force us to be so comprehensive in our treatment of the subject that the result would be unattractive to busy clinicians. These individuals are frequently several months behind in their reading of even journal articles so that books are not read but rather "put on the shelf for future reference."

Consequently, we decided on a middle ground, something between a journal article and a textbook. Fortunately, the editorial policy and goals of the Optometric Extension Program Foundation's Curriculum II were quite compatible with our intent and target audience.

Our next major decision related to content. We knew what we wanted to include, but had to then determine what we wanted to leave out. Our combined experience in clinically using standardized visual perceptual tests and teaching optometry students and practicing optometrists how to productively incorporate these tests into their diagnostic regimens was quite helpful here. As we state in the introduction, we confined the topics to those we believe the clinician "needs to know" to maximally apply these tests for effective and optimal patient management. You can determine how well you've mastered these topics by taking the Self Assessment Test at the end of this monograph (p.47).

Further, in the interest of orienting the reader, there is another concept that was influential in shaping this monograph. In the minds of many, the subject area of Tests and Measurements is synonymous with research design and statistics. We feel it quite important to state at the outset that this is not so. Although Tests and Measurements and sound clinical research are based in clearly stated and logical methodology, and share some of the same statistics, the individual who is well versed in clinical research is not, a priori, an expert in Tests and Measurements and vice versa. But since virtually all scientifically based investigations must utilize some form of Tests and Measurements, the person who masters the contents of this manual will find that he or she has also become a more sophisticated reader of clinical research.

Finally, we want to strongly recommend a way to read this monograph so that the included concepts and topics become as meaningful as possible. The reader should obtain the manual that accompanies a test of visual perception and reports the test design, standardization process, norms, and other statistics. As each section or topic area in this monograph is completed, the reader should find the discussion and data in the manual for the particular topic and compare the one to the other. While the manual for any test can be used in this manner, we'd suggest obtaining that from either the Test of Visual Perceptual Skills or the Developmental Test of Visual Motor Integration, since most of the topic areas we will cover are included in these manuals. Both of these tests are listed in the Appendix (p. 59).

INTRODUCTION

Conscious consideration of statistical concepts and test design usually plays a minor role in the day-to-day activities of most health care practitioners. Standard deviations, standard scores, percentiles and test validity are recalled as concepts once learned but soon forgotten and of limited use in the management of patients. In reality, however, statistical concepts are basic to sound clinical thinking. Virtually all areas of diagnosis and intervention depend on whether the findings are "within normal limits" or whether the intervention is effective in significantly changing numerical findings associated with the patient's performance and/or behavior.

This is particularly true for optometrists who treat patients with visual functional disorders. A diagnosis is made, for example, by comparing a patient's symptoms or performance deficits to the expected measurements of accommodation, vergences, eye movements and perceptual tests. Preventive care also is based on deviations from expected findings.

Consequently, the clinician, who truly understands the basics of test design, practices at a more enlightened level than one who has little appreciation of these concepts. Utilizing this knowledge enables the optometrist to be aware of the limitations and the strengths of clinical tests, and the patient is the ultimate beneficiary.

There is still another important reason for the clinician

to understand and apply the concepts of tests and measurements. This relates to enhanced professional communication. When treating children who have functional and/or learning disorders, optometrists frequently interact with members of other professions because of the interdisciplinary nature of these disorders. They include educators, clinical psychologists, neuropsychologists, pediatricians, and occupational and physical therapists. These practitioners communicate among themselves and with other involved professionals in a common language. It is a language that quantifies performance and behavior in terms of means, scaled scores, percentiles, and other statistical measures. The benefit is that communication is facilitated, because the language is clear and available to all. A bridge between the professions is there for all who wish to use it. Only recently have optometrists begun to take advantage of this opportunity, and the results have been quite good.

Further, optometrists often find it important to measure the difference in behavior of an individual who is performing the same task at different times. Common examples are retesting a patient after a few days to be certain whether a deficit in visual memory actually exists, or testing a child before and after perceptual therapy in order to establish that significant improvement in, for example, figure-ground skills has indeed taken place. There are also occasions when the optometrist is interested in comparing the performance of two different patients. If, for example, patient A, an average reader, completes the Six Figure Divided Form Board[1,2] more rapidly than patient B, a poor reader, it is of interest to know whether the difference in time to complete the task is indeed a meaningful distinction. Other times, it is of special concern to determine whether a statistically significant difference exists in a particular patient between visual memory and visual sequential memory, two related skills. As the reader will see, a difference in raw scores between two tests is not always indicative of a real difference in performance. Since optometrists are involved in measuring a wide range of visual behavioral and cognitive skills, these comparisons are helpful in arriving at a valid diagnosis and/or treatment plan.

In this monograph, the authors have an overall goal of reviewing some of the basic measurement concepts necessary to understand and evaluate the design and statistics of clinical tests. We will be referring to a number of clinical probes frequently used by behavioral optometrists. They are individually referenced in the text when appropriate and/or are also listed according to sources in the appendix on page 59. A more specific goal is to enable the reader to productively apply these concepts. Consequently, the practitioner's clinical testing program will be more meaningful, and patient care will be enhanced.

We have purposely limited our choice of test and measurement topics to those the clinician "needs to know." Only the basic aspects of these topics have been covered. For readers who wish to pursue these subjects in greater depth, we recommend the following sources:

1. Anastasi A. Psychological testing. 6th ed. New York:MacMillan Publ, 1988.

2. Guilford JP, Fruchter B. Fundamental statistics in psychology and education. 6th ed. New York:McGraw-Hill, 1978.

3. Munro BH, Visintainer MA, Page EB. Statistical methods for health care research. Philadelphia: J.B. Lippincott, 1986.

TEST
STANDARDIZATION

The term *test* requires careful attention. For the purpose of this monograph, *a test is an objective and standardized measure of a sample of behavior.*[3] Objective refers to measurements where judgment is minimized. That is, every trained observer of a performance ideally should arrive at precisely the same result. The time it takes a child to complete the Grooved Peg Board[2] or the number of digits correctly reported on the Tachistoscopic Exposure Test[2] are examples of objective measurements. On the other hand, the patient's report of first blur on the Positive Relative Accommodation Test (PRA) is considered subjective. There is no intent to imply that subjective responses and impressions obtained while observing the patient are not valuable sources of clinical information. Although impressionistic observations often allow the examiner to gain valuable information about the patient's problem-solving strategies, it should be kept in mind that if the behavior exists, it exists in some amount. If it exists in some amount, it can be measured. The seasoned clinician maximally utilizes both objective measurements and subjective observations of patient performance.

Standardized refers to uniformity of procedure. When a test is standardized, procedures, instrumentation, and scoring have been specified so that all conditions can be duplicated at different times and places. Consequently, the prescribed testing materials are used in each administration, and the instructions to the patients do not vary. Time limits should be carefully observed if they are stipulated. Sometimes, however, the patient is permitted additional time to complete the test so that comparisons between timed and untimed scores can be made.

Sample of behavior is the first "sample" that we shall address. When the need to assess a particular behavior is indicated, a test is selected that allows the examiner to observe and measure this behavior. For example, if there is a clinical necessity to obtain a sample of a child's visuomotor skills, the optometrist may select the Developmental Test of Visual Motor Integration. The child's score and observations of various behaviors during the test allow the clinician to draw certain conclusions about the child's visuomotor skills. A similar process takes place when using the Grooved Peg Board, the Wold Copying Test, or measuring the range of fusion. Each of these assessments represents a sample of a particular behavior.

Standardization Sample is another "sample" which is a factor in standardizing and norming data. The population is the larger, but similarly constituted group, from which the standardization sample is drawn. The population does not extend indefinitely; it has boundaries. Consequently, if a test is designed for grade two children, the population might not comprise every category of grade two children. For example, it is often specified that mentally-disabled and emotionally-disturbed children are not included. The sample, on the other hand, refers to the group of persons actually tested. This standardization sample should be a representative cross-section of the population for which a test is designed.

OBTAINING NORMS

The *Raw Score* is our starting point. When we test a patient, the data obtained is the raw score. The raw score may be the number of seconds to complete the Grooved Peg Board Test, the number of responses correct on the Visual Memory Subtest of the Test of Visual Perceptual Skills, or the number of objects the child can recall in the correct order on the Object Sequence Test of the Detroit Test of Learning Aptitude. The total raw score is usually the sum of the correct responses on a particular test or sub-test. However, in some tests, the raw score is the number of errors rather than number correct as in the Gardner Reversal Frequency Tests.

A raw score by itself, however, provides limited clinically useful information. In order to become more meaningful, it must be compared to something. One method is to compare the raw score to the total number of items in the test. If Helen correctly answered 70 out of 100 items on a vocabulary test, we can establish a basic comparison. We now know how Helen's performance compared to the optimum, i.e., to answer all items correctly. It is more meaningful, however, to compare Helen's score to that of her classmates. This enables us to obtain a ranking of her performance.

One might think that it would be useful to compare her raw score of 70 in vocabulary to one of 50 on an arithmetic test in order to determine her relative strength in these two areas. However, even if both tests had 100 items, raw scores alone rarely allow us to do this. In this situation, arithmetic is more of a "classroom bound" subject, a limiting factor in learning, while vocabulary represents, to a much greater degree, a reflection of life experience. In general, the comparison of raw scores, per se, is of little value, since we often are dealing with "apples and oranges."

In order to use raw scores for ranking or comparison purposes, it is necessary to understand the concepts and empirical processes involved in transforming them into a more versatile statistic. The first step in this process is the development of norms.

A norm describes the performance distribution of some representative sample of the population on a particular standardized test. The composition of the sample must be clearly defined. Norms make it possible to interpret a raw score, since the raw score may be compared with the performance distribution of the standardization sample. Norms can also provide a direct comparison of an individual's performance on different tasks or tests.

There are two kinds of norms, prescriptive and descriptive. *Prescriptive norms* define what ought to be. The original OEP norms,[4] developed more than 60 years ago, are prescriptive. *Descriptive norms*, on the other hand, refer to actual measurements. They represent the results derived when a carefully defined representative population sample is measured using standardized procedures.

There are certain criteria associated with good norms:

1. The sample of the population must be correctly defined by the author of the test.

2. Sampling error must be kept to a minimum. If we

measure only a relatively small segment of the total population, different samples could yield different results. The uncertainty introduced by such variations in results from these different samples constitutes the sampling error.[5] Since a larger standardization sample is more representative of the total population, the sampling error will be smaller. A sample of 100 or more subjects is considered to be sufficiently large to minimize the sampling error for the testing customarily done in the optometric practice.

3. The sample must be representative of the patient population that the optometrist is testing (e.g. normal students, reading-disabled, etc.)

Once the norms meet these criteria and those that assure proper standardization procedures have been used, the next step is to examine the distribution of the norms in the population sample.

Norms as a Measure of Central Tendency

In a normal distribution, most people have scores near the center of the curve. There are three principal measures of the center point of the normal distribution: mean, median, and mode. These are referred to as measures of central tendency (see Figure 1).

1. *Mean*: This statistic is the arithmetic average of a number of scores (N). The mean is written as $\bar{X}$. When the sum of all the scores (ΣX) is divided by the number of scores (N), the mean ($\bar{X}$) is expressed as $\frac{\Sigma X}{N}$. Since all scores contribute to the calculation, the mean is sensitive to extreme scores.

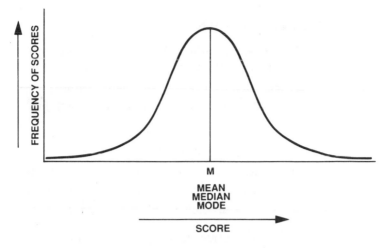

Figure 1. A bell-shaped curve of a perfect normal distribution; the mean, median and mode are coincident .

2. *Median:* The median is that point or score above and below which 50% of the group performs. It splits the frequency distribution in half: 50% of the scores are above the median, and 50% are below. As we shall see, it is by definition, the 50th percentile, P_{50} (p.17). Given a series of scores: 3, 9, 7, 1, 5, the median would be 5 since two scores are above 5 and two scores are below 5. Unlike the mean, the median is not affected by extreme scores.

3. *Mode:* The mode is the measurement value that has the highest frequency on a test. The mode usually is not a very useful statistic, although it is sometimes used in optometric research when we are interested in identifying a condition which is most frequently observed in the clinic. In a large sample, the mode is usually close to the mean and median and is not affected by extreme scores.

Scores in Terms of Variability

The next step is to determine how the individual raw scores vary about the mean. In an "ideal" normal distribution, the mean, median, and mode are the same value. (see Figure 1). There are several scores involved when discussing variability.

1. *Range:* The range is obtained by subtracting the lowest from the highest score and is the most easily calculated measure of variability. Since one score can have a large effect, statistically, it is quite crude.

2. *Deviation:* The difference between the raw score (X) and the mean ($\overline{X}$) is called the deviation score. Calculating it is a simple procedure. The deviation score (x) is expressed as

$$x = (X - \overline{X})$$

For example, let us suppose that John scores 20 on an arithmetic test (ar) and 50 on a spelling test (sp). If the mean for the arithmetic test is 15 and the mean for the spelling test is 60, then the two deviation scores, x_{ar} and x_{sp}, are (20 − 15 = +5) and (50 − 60 = −10) respectively.

3. *Standard Deviation:* This statistic provides a measure of how the individual scores are distributed about the mean in a normal bell-shaped distribution.

To obtain the standard deviation, all scores in the normative population are considered. The deviation score (x) is calculated for each raw score and squared. This eliminates negative quantities that would result when the raw score is less than the mean. Otherwise, the sum of the unsquared scores in a symmetrical normal distribution would equal zero. All of the individual squared deviations are then added (Σx^2) and the total is divided by the number of subjects ($\frac{\Sigma x^2}{N}$). The resulting quotient is called the variance[6] (s^2). The square root of this expression yields the most used, useful and meaningful statistic in tests and measurements, the *standard deviation* (s).

$$s=\sqrt{\frac{\Sigma x^2}{N}}$$

The numerical value of the standard deviation represents the average deviation score and defines the distribution of scores around the mean.

If we are using a test where the raw score indicates the number of correct answers, the numerical value of one standard deviation is added to the numerical value of the mean to obtain the precise value of one standard deviation above the mean (+1s). Scores that are between the mean and +1s are said to be within 1 standard deviation above the mean. If the numerical value of the standard deviation is subtracted from the mean, the precise value of one standard deviation below the mean (–1s) is obtained. Scores that are between the mean and –1s are said to lie within 1 standard deviation below the mean.

As is indicated in Figure 2 (page 12), approximately 34% of the normally distributed population used in the standardization of this hypothetical test scored within 1 standard deviation above the mean and an additional 34% scored within one standard deviation below the mean. Consequently, 68% of the population sample scored within the interval represented by ± 1 standard deviation from the mean.

The meaning and utility of ± 2 and 3 standard deviations may be similarly illustrated. When the numerical value

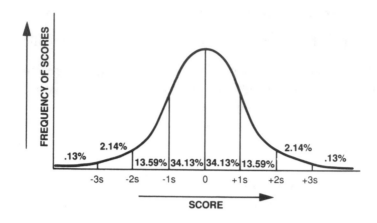

Figure 2. The exact percentages of the population falling within the various standard deviations is illustrated. In the text, these are numerically "rounded off."

of the standard deviation is doubled and then added to or subtracted from the mean, the precise values of 2 standard deviations above and below the mean can be determined respectively. Figure 2 shows the interval on the bell curve between 1 and 2 standard deviations is represented by an additional 14% of the subjects. Therefore the intervals between the mean and ± 2 standard deviations represent 34 + 14 times 2 or 96% of the subjects in a normal distribution. Almost 100% of the subjects are included in the range from +3 to –3 standard deviations. *The numerical value of the standard deviation remains constant although the percentage of population included in successive intervals decreases significantly.* Every score contributes to the standard deviation. Its value is not dependent upon a single score. When the scores are clustered closely about the mean, the standard deviation is small. When the scores are widely distributed, the standard deviation is large.

A basic understanding of the standard deviation allows the clinician to further quantify a patient's performance. For example, the patient attains a raw score of 12 in a test where the mean score for the individual's age is 16. With just this information the deviation score $(X - \bar{X})$ can be calculated and is -4. We know that the patient scored less than expected since a negative number results, but we do not know whether the performance is "bad" or "very bad." If the standard deviation is 2, the raw score is then 2 standard deviations below the mean, and is interpreted as "very bad." If instead, the standard deviation is 5, then the raw score (12) is within one standard deviation below the mean and can be considered as "bad" on our arbitrary scale.

While comparing the patient's deviation score to the standard deviation is admittedly a relatively gross comparison, it is more enlightening than just comparing the raw score to the mean. Essentially, it is a first step in obtaining a more precise interpretation of the raw score in a normal distribution. The standard deviation is one of the building blocks for obtaining derived scores. These allow us to further pinpoint a patient's performance and are covered in the next section.

DERIVED SCORES

A lthough an understanding of the statistical concept, standard deviation, allows us to compare a patient's performance to that of a standardized population in a way that is productive, the interpretation is too gross. To state that a child's score is "within one standard deviation below the mean" lacks specificity when comparing the score with the scores of other children. Is the child's performance slightly, moderately, or very much worse than his peers?

Once the clinician obtains a measure of the patient's raw score, there are a number of ways to interpret this data. The use of *within group norms*, for example, enables the examiner to compare the patient's performance with that of the standardization group. In order to understand various interpretations normally considered under the umbrella of within group norms, three statistical entities are discussed: z scores (including scaled and standard scores), percentiles and equivalent scores. The latter usually are called developmental norms and are discussed in the following chapter.

z scores are sometimes called standard scores. *The z score expresses the distance of an individual's raw score from the mean in terms of the standard deviation.* The z score is easily obtained. The raw score is subtracted from the mean $(X - \bar{X})$, and this deviation score is divided by the standard deviation:

$$z = \frac{(X - \overline{X})}{s}$$

When the raw score has the same value as the mean, the z score is zero. In Figure 3, assume that the numerical value of the mean is 12, and the standard deviation is 2. When the raw score equals the mean, 12, z equals 0. In a normal distribution, z always equals zero at the mean. On the other hand, if the raw score were equal to 14, one standard deviation above the mean, z would equal +1. Similarly, a raw score of 10 would have a z score of −1. *When the raw scores are normally distributed, the curve of a z score is a normal distribution with a mean of 0 and a standard deviation of 1.* Since the deviation score (numerator) and the standard deviation (denominator) are always in the same units, the units cancel out and yield a pure number. By converting raw scores of different tests to z scores, it is possible for the optometrist to compare a child's relative performances on tests that use different

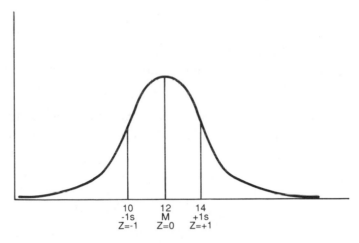

Figure 3. The mean (m) is 12 and the standard deviation(s) is 2. The relationship between the mean, standard deviation and z scores is indicated.

dimensions. Thus, the time (in seconds) to complete the Divided Form Board can be compared to the number of digits correct (span of perception) on the Tachistoscopic Exposure Test.

Usually, raw scores do not correspond to exact multiples of the deviation score, and, therefore, the z score most frequently is a decimal. In the above example, a raw score of 15 translates to z score of 1.50 ($\frac{15-12}{2}$). It becomes evident that if a test has a "near normal" distribution, and the mean and standard deviation are provided, the patient's raw score can easily be transformed into a z score. The z score specifies precisely how the patient performs in terms of standard deviation units.

The z score can be used to interpret the patient's performance in other ways, too. Table 1 makes it possible to convert z scores into percentiles. This statistic is familiar since psychologists and educators frequently report the results of students' tests in percentiles. *Percentiles measure the percentage of individuals in a standardized sample whose scores fall below a given raw score.*[3] Percentiles should not be confused with percentages. Percentages are based upon ratios, while percentiles depend upon the frequency distribution of the scores.

Percentiles do not represent a linear scale. For example, the increment in raw score between the 6th and 16th percentile is greater than the increment between the 40th and 50th percentile. Inspection of Figure 1 shows that in a bell-shaped curve, the frequency of the scores is greater near the center, causing the scores to be clustered closer together. Finally, because they are non-linear, percentiles cannot be added, subtracted, multiplied, or divided. However, they are easy to understand and are universally applicable.

TABLE 1

z Score	Percentile		z Score	Percentile	
	+z	-z		+z	-z
0.00	50	50	1.50	93	7
0.05	52	48	1.55	94	6
0.10	54	46	1.60	95	5
0.15	56	44	1.65	95	5
0.20	58	42	1.70	96	4
0.25	60	40	1.75	96	4
0.30	62	38	1.80	96	4
0.35	64	36	1.85	97	3
0.40	66	34	1.90	97	3
0.45	67	33	1.95	97	3
0.50	69	31	2.00	98	2
0.55	71	29	2.05	98	2
0.60	73	27	2.10	98	2
0.65	74	26	2.15	98	2
0.70	76	24	2.20	99	1
0.75	77	23	2.25	99	1
0.80	79	21	2.30	99	1
0.85	80	20	2.35	99	1
0.90	82	18	2.40	99	1
0.95	83	17	2.45	99	1
1.00	84	16	2.50	99	1
1.05	85	15	2.55	99.5	0.5
1.10	86	14	2.60	99.5	0.5
1.15	87	13	2.65	99.6	0.4
1.20	88	12	2.70	99.6	0.4
1.25	89	11	2.75	99.7	0.3
1.30	90	10	2.80	99.7	0.3
1.35	91	9	2.85	99.8	0.2
1.40	92	8	2.90	99.8	0.2
1.45	93	7	2.95	99.8	0.2
			3.00	99.9	0.1

Table 1. Conversion of z scores to percentiles.

The symmetrical bell-shaped curve of the population sample in Figure 4 (page 18) illustrates the relationship between the mean, standard deviation, z score, and percentile. Since the median (line z = 0) "splits" the curve, it represents the 50th percentile (P_{50}). As stated earlier, ± 1 standard deviation each encompasses 34% of the population under the curve. Consequently, +1 standard deviation is the 84th percentile (P84) since it accounts for 34% more of the population than P50. Because it represents 34% less of the population than P50, −1 standard deviation is at the 16th percentile.

There is often some ambiguity in the interpretation of "one standard deviation below the mean." The researcher, on the one hand, seeks to identify a population of subjects whose findings are undoubtedly poor. Those falling below the 16th percentile are deemed to be in this category. This kind of reasoning is often applied when biological functions are assessed; laboratory findings within -1s are frequently characterized as being within the low normal range. However, in performance testing that is being used to measure an individual's visual functional and/or perceptual skills, this type of reasoning can be misleading. Any score below the 50th percentile is suspect, especially when a child's IQ is average or better, since the criterion is mastery of the task. Scores below

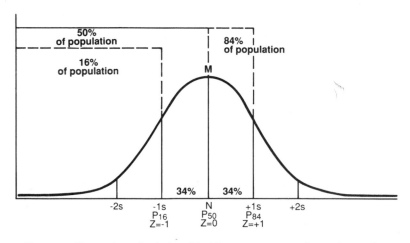

Figure 4. Illustration of relationships between percentiles, +1 standard deviations and z scores.

-0.5s, the 31st percentile, should be considered poor and represent a real dysfunction in a task or subject area.

The z scores also form the basis of *scaled scores*. The behavioral optometrist frequently receives scaled scores, especially when reading reports concerning IQs and other educational tests. For example, the results of the subtests of the Wechsler Intelligence Test for Children-Revised (WISC-R)[7] are recorded as scaled scores. When a test has a number of homogeneous subtests, scaled scores enable the examiner to readily compare strengths and weaknesses in a number of areas. *Each subtest is arbitrarily assigned a mean of ten and a standard deviation of 3.* The scale scores are calculated directly from the z scores for each age group using the following expression:

Scaled Score = 10 + 3z

When a child's raw score in a subtest is the same as the mean for a particular age range in the normative population, then $z - 0$ since $X-\overline{X} - 0$. The scaled score is 10, and it, too, is at the mean or P_{50}. On the other hand, if a child's scaled score is 13 on the Coding Subtest and 6 on the Block Design Subtest of the WISC-R, then it is evident that he is scoring one standard deviation above the mean in Coding and within two standard deviations below the mean in Block Design.

The z score is also used in calculating the *Standard Score*, although other names such as Deviation IQ and Perceptual Quotient are used. Standard scores are used to express the performance level on tests that have no subtests, such as the Developmental Test of Visual Motor Integration (VMI) or in assessment instruments that have subtests, such as the Test of Visual Perceptual Skills (TVPS) in order to determine the total battery score.

In tests used by optometrists, most frequently the Standard Score is assigned a mean of 100 and a standard deviation of 15. It is calculated as follows:

Standard Score = 100 + 15z

When using the VMI, the patient's raw score can be converted to a standard score by means of the tables provided in the test manual. For the TVPS and other test batteries that are comprised of a number of separate homogeneous subtests, the standard score is used only when all of the subtest scores are available. This type of standard score is sometimes called Perceptual Quotient. In these instances, the sum of all the subtest scores is obtained and converted to a standard score and percentiles using the tables provided in the manual. Table 2 is used for this purpose in the TVPS.

We now turn our attention to another group of norms that are derived somewhat differently, developmental norms.

TABLE 2

TABLE 20. Conversion of Sum of Scaled Scores to Perceptual Quotients and Percentile Ranks.

Sum	PQ	Rank	Sum	PQ	Rank	Sum	PQ	Rank	Sum	PQ	Rank
128+	160+	99+	73	103	58	45	74	4	17	45	1-
128	160	99+	72	102	55	44	73	4	16	44	1-
127	159	99+	71	101	53	43	72	3	15	43	1-
126	158	99+	70	100	50	42	71	3	14	42	1-
125	157	99+	69	99	47	41	70	2	13	41	1-
124	156	99+	68	98	45	40	69	2	12	40	1-
123	155	99+	67	97	42	39	68	2	12-	40-	1-
122	154	99+	66	96	39	38	67	1			
121	153	99+	65	95	37	37	66	1			
120	152	99+	64	94	34	36	65	1			
119	151	99+	63	93	32	35	64	1			
118	150	99+	62	92	30	34	63	1			
117	149	99+	61	91	27	33	62	1			
116	148	99+	60	90	25	32	61	1-			
115	147	99+	59	89	23	31	60	1-			
114	146	99+	58	88	21	30	58	1-			
113	145	99+	57	87	19	29	57	1-			
112	144	99+	56	85	16	28	56	1-			
111	143	99+	55	84	14	27	55	1-			
110	142	99+	54	83	13	26	54	1-			
109	140	99+	53	82	12	25	53	1-			
108	139	99+	52	81	10	24	52	1-			
107	138	99	51	80	9	23	51	1-			
106	137	99	50	79	8	22	50	1-			
105	136	99	49	78	7	21	49	1-			
104	135	99	48	77	6	20	48	1-			
103	134	99	47	76	5	19	47	1-			
102	133	99	46	75	5	18	46	1-			

Reproduced from the Test of Visual Perceptual Skills with permission from Psychological and Educational Publications, Inc., Burlingame, Calif.

DEVELOPMENTAL NORMS

In optometry, as in psychology and education, it is sometimes appropriate to evaluate an aspect of the child's development with the expected for his age, grade, or some other parameter. The yardsticks are developmental norms, and although they do not lend themselves well to precise statistical treatment, they are descriptive and clinically useful. Four types of developmental norms are discussed.

1. *Age equivalent:* This measure represents the raw score (RS) that is statistically characteristic of a particular age in the normative sample for a given task. That is, the age equivalent represents the mean or median raw score obtained on a test by children of a specific chronological age (CA). In practice, the examiner obtains the raw score of a child and refers to the table of norms in the test manual in order to determine the age equivalent. The latter is usually listed as, e.g., 5 years, 3 months, or simply 5-3. Age equivalents provide a quick estimation of performance by comparing the child's chronological age to the age equivalent. Table 3 illustrates how the raw score is converted to an Age Equivalent Score in the TVPS. In this test it is termed "Perceptual Age."

TABLE 3

TABLE 19. Conversion of Raw Scores to Visual-Perceptual Ages.

RS	VD	VM	VSR	VFC	VSM	VFG	VC	RS
16			>12-11		>12-11			16
15	>12-11		12-8		11-1			15
14	11-8	>12-11	9-8	>12-11	10-0	>12-11		14
13	9-7	11-1	8-0	12-1	8-10	11-9	>12-11	13
12	8-2	9-7	7-2	10-2	8-2	9-10	11-8	12
11	7-5	8-7	6-7	9-0	7-8	8-10	10-4	11
10	6-9	7-8	6-1	8-1	7-4	8-0	9-6	10
9	6-3	7-0	5-10	7-6	7-0	7-5	8-10	9
8	5-10	6-5	5-6	7-0	6-9	6-11	8-2	8
7	5-6	5-11	5-2	6-6	6-6	6-5	7-6	7
6	5-2	5-5	4-10	5-11	6-2	6-1	6-10	6
5	4-10	5-1	4-7	5-5	5-10	5-8	6-2	5
4	4-6	4-8	4-4	4-11	5-7	5-3	5-7	4
3	4-2	4-2	4-1	4-5	4-11	4-10	4-11	3
2	<4-0	<4-0	<4-0	<4-0	4-1	4-5	4-4	2
1					<4-0	4-1	<4-0	1
0						<4-0		0

Reproduced from the Test of Visual Perceptual Skills with permission from Psychological and Educational Publications, Inc., Burlingame, Calif.

While clinically useful, age equivalents are subject to the non-linear characteristics of a child's development. This is especially evident in motor development tasks, where, for example, development of certain skills is much more rapid from 5 to 6 years than from 7 to 8 years. It is therefore difficult to establish what constitutes markedly poorer behavior. The clinician who uses only age equivalents in his assessment runs the risk of either over- or under-estimating the significance of scores that are above or below those that correspond to the child's chronological age.

2. *Mental Age*: This concept is similar to the age equivalent norms except that mental age (MA) tests deal with various aspects of mental development. The questions address areas of knowledge which customarily improve with age, such as vocabulary, mental arithmetic, general information and reasoning. Mental age is obtained by comparing a child's score with norms established from a population of children of the same age. If a 7-year-old child does as well as the average 8-year-old, his mental age is said to be 8 years. Mental age has different meaning at different ages. For example, one year of mental growth from age 3 to 4 is equivalent to three years of growth at ages 9 to 12 since intellectual development progresses more rapidly at younger ages. Although the concept of mental age is still clinically useful, in practice the ratio, MA/CA (CA is the chronological age) is not used directly for the measurement of intelligence. The most commonly used assessment, the Wechsler Intelligence Test for Children - Revised (WISC-R), consists of verbal and performance batteries, and, as was discussed, they are expressed as standard scores.

3. *Grade Equivalents:* These commonly used norms compare an individual's performance with the average student's performance in a particular grade in each subject. Grade equivalent (GE) scores for a test are calculated by finding the mean raw score, the 50th percentile, of the standardization sample for each grade level. The procedure is similar to determining age norms, except a 10-month school year is used. Therefore, if the average number of correct answers on a vocabulary test for grade 4 in September is 30, then 30 correct answers represent grade 4.1 since September is the first month of grade 4. If the average number correct at the beginning of grade 3 is 20 correct, then 20 represents grade 3.1. Intermediate scores, when not directly measured, may be obtained by interpolation.

Although GE scores have popular appeal since they are easy to explain, there are a number of caveats. Grade equivalents, like other norms, are based on normal distributions. Therefore, if a score is near the low end or the high end of the range of the test, one or two additional correct answers can vary the GE score by as much as two years. However, if the examiner selects a test level that places the "low end" child between the mean (50th percentile) and −1s (16th percentile), GEs may be very helpful in measuring improvement from supplementary instruction. This may require, for example, that a third grade test be used for a child in grade 4.

Some subjects such as arithmetic are relatively more "classroom-bound" than others such as reading. That is, most children generally do not learn long division or adding fractions by themselves. Consequently, a child could have a higher reading grade equivalent than arithmetic but be in a higher percentile in arithmetic than reading. Further, GEs can be misleading. A grade-4 child whose June arithmetic score is 6.9 is not necessarily prepared to do grade 7 arithmetic. It just means that the student is a very bright 4th-grader. Finally, the benchmark of the GE is the "average child," the 50th percentile child, who often represents the "C" student.

4. *Developmental Stage Norms:* These are also called *ordinal* norms, and they are designed to identify the *order* in which the child reaches successive stages in the development of specific behavioral functions. They are based on either a proposed or proven hierarchy in the development of a skill or behavior such as locomotion and motor, speech and language, emotion, and concept formation. The ordinality also refers to the orderly progression from stage to stage in the normal development of each individual. Although each major stage carries with it an age range in recognition of individual variability in child development, the emphasis is on the qualitative descriptions of the child's behavior.

An example familiar to optometrists is Piaget's stages of cognitive development. He divided intellectual development into four stages: Sensorimotor Period (birth to 2 years); Preoperational Period (2 to 7 years); Period of Concrete Operations (7 to 11 years); Period of Formal Operations (11 to 15 years).[8] Piaget contended that although the sequence of these periods is fixed and the same for all children, in normal development, different children progress from one stage to the next at somewhat different ages. Each stage presupposes a mastery of prerequisite behavior that is characteristic of an earlier stage.[9] The utility of this type of scale is that it provides the practitioner and parent with an overview of the progression of the child's development. Since the developmental stages follow in a constant order, it at once provides knowledge of where the child is now, where he was, and where he is going.

RELIABILITY

The previous sections provide the clinician with a basis for judging whether or not the expectations of sound test design are met. The nature and character of the standardization process, and the development of norms in terms of central tendency and variability have been discussed. Within group norms have been compared to developmental norms. All of these statistics are highly dependent upon the integrity of the test in terms of its repeatability. The generic term for this measurement is *reliability*. The need for consistency in measurement is of paramount importance for clinical testing.

When utilizing a particular test, the clinician should be confident that he is obtaining a true measure of the patient's performance. In other words, if the test, itself, or an alternate equivalent version is administered the next day or the next week, how closely will the results compare to the original test score?

Comparing or "co-relating" the scores of a group of individuals when the test is administered on two successive occasions is one method of obtaining the reliability of a test. The relationship, or correlation, of the two sets of measurements is known as the *reliability coefficient* and is expressed as r_{tt}. The reliability coefficient is the coefficient of correlation between the first and second administration of the test. The factors that comprise r_{tt} include the mean score and standard deviation for each administration, the number of subjects, and the sum of the deviation scores of each of the subjects on the two tests. The Pearson product-moment coefficient of correlation[6] is the most frequently used procedure.

If the individual who obtained the lowest score on the first administration of the test also obtained the lowest score on the second, and the same rank order was observed for every other subject who took the test, r_{tt} would be equal to 1, a perfect correlation. In practice, this is not likely to happen. Usually, in optometric testing, a reliability coefficient of .8 is acceptable. There are other uses of correlation such as determining the degree of association between accommodative facility and the length of time an individual can read comfortably, and this aspect will be covered later (see page 38).

Error Variance

Ideally, as stated above, if the same or equivalent test is administered under standardized conditions to the same population sample, the correlation between the two tests should be 1. Since this is not the case, there must be some differences in the test scores.

What are the sources of these differences?[10] A change in attitude or degree of attention in a child between test administrations often can be the cause. Other examples include environmental variations such as noise, temperature, and ventilation in a room. The effect of these factors that are difficult, if not impossible, to control is a change in the individual's score from one test administration to the next. The cumulative effect of this phenomenon on the total group is a different standard deviation, and the normal curve becomes flatter or steeper depending upon whether the standard deviation increases or decreases, respectively. It is this difference in variance that concerns us. The use of the term "Error" variance is misleading since the difference in performance, either individually or cumulatively, is not an error. Actually, it is a recognition that there are chance factors which effect the total performance.

In practice, we can obtain the percent of error variance by subtracting the obtained correlation between the two administrations of the test, the reliability coefficient (r_{tt}), from a perfect correlation, 1. The percent of error variance is inversely related to the reliability and can be expressed mathematically by the following formula:

$$\textbf{Percent of Error Variance} = (1 - r_{tt}) \cdot 100$$

Therefore, when the reliability is .8, it follows that 80% of the total variance is true variance and the error variance is .2, or 20%. As the reliability of a test increases, the percent of error variance decreases. The importance of error variance will become more evident in the discussion of Standard Error of Measurement (see pages 32-36).

How Reliability is Measured

There are a number of ways to measure reliability, and each addresses a slightly different aspect of error variance. In each method, however, the results of one set of measurements are correlated with the second to determine the reliability.

1. *Test - retest* Since the same test is used in each administration, the contents of the test remain the same and do not contribute to the error variance. However, a time interval does exist. Therefore, we are securing a measure of the extent to which the score may be generalized over time. This is an important

consideration to optometrists when treating binocular and perceptual dysfunctions.

2. *Equivalent form* In educational and perceptual testing, sometimes alternate forms of a test are available. Instead of providing the same test again, an alternate, but equivalent test is administered. This approach involves two types of error variance: time and content. We assume, of course, that the two forms are parallel. That is, the content is similar in difficulty, and there are the same number of items. The form of the test should remain the same (e.g., multiple choice). The standardization procedures should be identical, and the sample of population the same. As in the test - retest, the possibility of a learning experience exists because of the two test administrations.

3. *Split half* The final alternative involves a single administration of one test. By dividing the test items into comparable halves using odd and even numbered responses, two separate scores can be obtained. Using an odd/even split solves the problem of accounting for the increasing difficulty of items often found in tests. There is a small content error and no time error variance when using one administration of a single test. Fatigue and practice considerations are also avoided. The odd/even split, however, reduces the effective number of items in each test in half, and, therefore, the test's author must apply a special formula to compensate for this discrepancy.

Before using a test, the optometrist should read the portion of the instruction manual which discusses reliability. Reliability is usually lower for younger children and children who perform more poorly since guessing and poor concentration are likely to influence the results to a greater extent. To improve reliability in a test, more items may be added. Each item then carries less weight. The lower the reliability, the more difficult it is for the examiner to determine what can be inferred from the test results. Next we shall see how reliability can effect the interpretation of individual scores.

Standard Error of Measurement (SEM)

The standard error of measurement (SEM) is the application of measurement and error variance to the test score of an individual. The concept of error variance has established that there may be a difference in the score of a test upon remeasurement. *The SEM provides us with a reasonable estimate of the amount or range of fluctuation that we may expect in an individual's score.* The amount of this "error" depends upon the standard deviation and the reliability, the same factors which contributed to error variance.

The SEM is also useful to the clinician in those situations when standardized pre- and post-therapy testing is done. It enables the tester to determine whether the difference between the test scores that assessed the particular visual skill being treated is (1) within the expected range of fluctuation or (2) is truly an improvement that has resulted from therapy.

By using the equation

$$SEM = s \ \sqrt{1 - r_{tt}}$$

the standard error of measurement can be calculated (s is standard deviation, and $1- r_{tt}$ is the error variance). For example, if r_{tt} for the Six Figure Divided Form Board were .89, and the standard deviation 15 seconds then the SEM would be: $(15) \ \sqrt{1 - .89} = 5$. We could alternately retest a single subject 100 times, calculate the mean and find the standard deviation of the 100 scores. This standard deviation would be the SEM, and it would represent the standard deviation of the distribution of the 100 scores around the obtained mean.

Thus, if an obtained score on a test is 50, and the SEM is 5, we can conclude that the true score lies between 45 and 55. Further, we can predict that if the subject is retested, 68% of the time (which is the range of ±1 standard deviation) the new score will be between 45 and 55. For the remaining 32% of the time the SEM will exceed this range. If we wish to be more conservative the following rules of thumb apply:

1. To further increase the accuracy of the obtained test score to the 85% level of confidence, multiply the SEM by 1.44. In the above case (1.44 x 5), the product is 7. The expected range of test scores is now 50 ± 7. We can now predict that the obtained score, upon retesting, will fall within the range of 43 to 57 some 85% of the time.

2. Similarly, the 95%, or .05 level of confidence is determined by multiplying the SEM by 1.96 (5 x 1.96) which yields a range from 40 to 60 (50 ±10) in the above example.

The SEM therefore, provides the optometrist with a better understanding of the significance and boundaries of the tests she is administering and the therapy she will render.

The SEM is also used when we want to know whether a patient is performing better in one skill or another. Here, the *difference* between two scores is being compared. In the case of the TVPS, we may wish to know whether there is a significant difference between the Visual Memory (VM) and the Visual Sequential Memory (VSM) scaled scores. Either of the following equivalent equations enables the examiner to make this determination. If the author of the test provides the SEM, equation 1 is used. On the other hand, equation 2 is used when the standard deviation and reliability, but not the SEM, are supplied.

Equation 1: $SEM_{dif} = \sqrt{(SEM_1)^2 + (SEM_2)^2}$

Equation 2: $SEM_{dif} = s\sqrt{2 - r_{11} - r_{22}}$

r_{11} and r_{22} are the reliabilities of each test. The standard deviations of the two tests are the same since scaled scores are used in the TVPS.

If we are using the TVPS with an 8-year-old child, the reliability of the visual memory subtest (VM) is .74, and the reliability of the visual sequential memory subtest (VSM) is .86. Since we are working with scaled scores, the standard deviation(s) is always 3. By substituting these findings in Equation 2, we find that the SEM_{dif} equals 1.9 which, clinically, is 2. *We now know that the scaled score of one test must differ from the other by at least 2 in order for the scores to be considered significantly different.* That is, if testing VM results in a scaled score of 7, then VSM must show a scaled score of at least 9 to be considered significantly better.

Still another use of the SEM_{dif} is when we want to compare a particular skill before and after vision therapy. The question here is whether an improvement in the score following vision therapy is real or merely a function of the error of measurement (SEM). In other words, how much improvement in the score is necessary so that we are confident that the change in score is the result of the therapy and not spurious.

Equation 2 is the starting point to answer this question. However, since we are using the same test to obtain both the pre- and post-therapy scores, r_{11} and r_{22} are identical. With this in mind, equation 2 now becomes:

$$SEM_{dif} = s \sqrt{2 - 2r_{11}}$$

By factoring out $\sqrt{2}$, the equation now becomes:

$$SEM_{dif} = \sqrt{2} \cdot s \sqrt{1 - r_{11}}$$

and since: $s \sqrt{1 - r_{11}} = 1$ SEM

then:

Equation 3: $SEM_{dif} = \sqrt{2} \cdot SEM$

Equation 3 represents the minimum difference required between pre- and post-therapy scores for the 68% level of confidence. To obtain the 85% level of confidence it is necessary to multiply equation 3 by 1.44. Since 1.44 is very close to the value of the square root of 2 (which is 1.41), we can compute the 85% level of confidence as follows:

Equation 4: $SEM_{dif} = 1.44 \cdot \sqrt{2} \cdot SEM = 2$ SEM

The clinician who is involved in vision therapy should keep Equation 4 in mind when considering the efficacy of the intervention being rendered. For example, if the scaled scores on a test improved from 6 prior to therapy to 8 following therapy, the improvement would not meet the 85% criterion if the SEM were 1.5 (2 x 1.5 = 3). In fact, the results would barely meet the 68% requirements: 1.41 x 1.5 = 2.1 (Equation 3). Figure 5 (page 36) graphically illustrates why the 85% level of confidence (2SEM) is the yardstick used to determine the validity of an improvement in score following therapy.

Consequently, when testing a particular child, the SEM is of more practical value than simply knowing the reliability of a test. An understanding of the SEM enables the optometrist to improve the precision of his/her diagnosis and be more confident about the results of the therapy administered to patients.

WHY 2SEM?

(A) Pre- $\overline{5\quad 7\quad 9}$ SEM=2

(B) Post- $\overline{7\quad 9\quad 11}$ 2SEM=4

Before therapy, the patient's raw score was 7 on a test with an SEM of 2. This is graphically illustrated in (A). After therapy, the score improves to 9, as illustrated in (B). Although the post-therapy obtained score is 9, it is possible that the true score is 7 (9-2), and no real improvement resulted. The range of confidence changed from 5 to 9, to 7 to 11. In order for the clinician to be certain that the improvement in performance is truly the result of the therapy, the gain must be ≥ 2 SEM (i.e., ≥ 11) since 8 and 9 fit into the pre- and post-therapy ranges of confidence.

(C) Pre- $\overline{5\quad 7\quad 9}$

(D) Post- $\overline{\quad 9\quad 11\quad 13}$

On the other hand, in (C) and (D) an improvement of 4 units after therapy (2SEM) virtually eliminates overlap between pre- and post-therapy confidence ranges.

Figure 5

Importance of Reliability

In concluding the section, there are several important concepts to keep in mind concerning reliability and errors of measurement.

1. In order for a specific measurement (e.g., near phoria) to be clinically useful, the implicit measurement error must be known. Repeatability of a finding is a basic clinical requirement.

2. If the measurement error is too great, it is not possible to know whether or not your treatment is successful. If the measurement error is numerically close to the degree of improvement after the treatment, the "improvement" may be misleading.

3. High levels of reliability imply that standardized procedures were used in establishing the norms. When the exact testing procedures are not used in successive administrations of a test, it is unlikely that there will be a high level of repeatability in the results.

4. Reliability should be reported separately, in yearly intervals for the standardization sample (e.g., for age 5, 6, etc.). Calculating reliability across the entire standardization sample overestimates reliability since the number of subjects (N) is artificially inflated. When the N is greater, a single individual's score becomes less significant in the total group.[5]

When reliability is not given in a published test, presume that it was not measured. If the SEM is not provided, it may be calculated from the reliability and standard deviation.

CORRELATION

The reliability coefficient (see page 28) is just one application of correlation. In general, the coefficient of correlation defines the degree of association between two sets of data. For example, on the TVPS, the scaled scores on the Spatial Relations Subtest of a third grade class may be correlated with reading scores. Do the children who are better readers score better on this subtest while those who are poorer readers score lower?

Correlations may vary from 0 to +1 and −1. Zero represents no relationship. As the correlation increases toward either +1 or −1, the relationship improves toward a maximum. A correlation of +1 indicates a direct relationship such as the higher the near vergence findings, the longer individuals may be expected to read comfortably. An inverse relationship may be equally predictive. For example, the *less time* a kindergarten child takes to complete the Divided Form Board, the *higher* is his reading readiness score. Therefore, when the absolute correlation (omitting + and −) between the two scores is greater, the correspondence between the two sets of scores is greater.

Statistical significance and *percent of variance* are two other factors which are important for the clinician to understand.[5] A correlation of .6 represents a reasonably strong relationship between the two variables, X and Y ($r_{xy} = .6$). A weaker correlation would be $r_{xy} = .3$. Given the appropriate number of subjects, either of the correlations could be statistically significant. As the number of subjects is increased, the size of the correlation coefficient between two variables required for statistical significance is smaller.

Significance represents the probability that:

(1) the true correlation between two variables is zero and

(2) the obtained correlation is simply due to a sampling error, i.e. due to chance.

This information may be secured from a statistical table entitled "Significance levels for the Pearson product-moment coefficient of correlation."[5] Significance levels of .05 and lower (e.g., .01, .005) are usually acceptable although some conservative investigators require at least .01. If, for example, the obtained correlation is $r_{xy} = .6$ and the level of significance is $p<.001$, we may conclude: "The probability that the true correlation between the variables, X and Y, is zero is less than 1 chance in a 1000." Similarly, the obtained correlation $r_{xy} = .3$ may be significant at the .05 level. In this instance, the probability that the true correlation is zero is less than 5 chances in 100 ($p<.05$). In either case it should be remembered that the correlation provides us with the relationship between two variables, X and Y. It does not necessarily imply a cause and effect relationship between X and Y.

There are also a few other caveats:

1. A correlation of .50 is not twice as strong as a correlation of .25 nor does it represent a 50% probability.

2. An increment from .45 to .65 in correlation is not the same as an increase from .70 to .90. The increase from .70 to .90 is reflective of a stronger interaction between the variables.

3. A correlation of +.50 represents the same degree of association as -.50.

4. If a correlation is not significant or barely significant, the results should not be dismissed. Perhaps a larger sample or a slight change in methodology would increase the correlation.

A very practical interpretation of correlation is found in *percent of variance*. Also known as *Coefficient of Determination,* percent of variance is the coefficient of correlation squared (r^2) and multiplied by 100:

If $r_{xy} = .6$, then $r^2_{xy} = .36$, and $.36 \times 100 = 36\%$.

It is not difficult to obtain the percent of variance. Percent of variance is interpreted as follows: 36% of the variations in the dependent variable, Y, may be accounted for by variations in the independent variable, X. In a study by Solan, Mozlin, and Rumpf, [1] several perceptual findings were compared with total reading readiness at the end of kindergarten. The results were:

$R_{xy} = +.737$; $p < .0001$; $R^2 = .543$; Var = 54.3%

(When more than one experimental test variable (X_1, X_2, X_3) is compared to the criterion variable (Y), the coefficient of correlation is written as R_{xy}.)

They were able to conclude that the obtained coefficient of correlation between the perceptual tasks (X_1, X_2, X_3) which were the independent variables, and total readiness (Y), the dependent variable, was R = +.737, a strong positive correlation which was significant at p<.0001. The probability that the true correlation was zero was less than one chance in ten thousand. Fifty-four percent of the variations in total readiness could be accounted for by variations in perceptual skills.

On the other hand, a correlation of +.3 may be statistically significant, but since $r^2 = .09$, the percent of variance is only 9%. This means that 91% of the variations in the dependent variable are *not accounted for* by the independent variable(s). This type of information can be very useful in terms of guiding the clinician in arriving at a prognosis regarding specific effects of vision therapy. For example, if the r^2 between a test of visual discrimination and a reading test is 49%, it tells us that almost 50% of the variations in the reading scores can be accounted for by the skills measured on the visual discrimination test. Consequently, chances are that if the child's visual discrimination can be enhanced, it will have a favorable effect on reading. On the other hand, if the r^2 between the same two variables was 9%, the impact of vision therapy to improve visual discrimination probably would have a minimal effect on the child's reading performance. The percent of variance provides us with a measure of the usefulness of the correlation. That is, how meaningful are the results? With this information in mind, let us now consider validity.

VALIDITY

Validity is a particularly important concept for behavioral optometrists. Since those who treat children often administer a diverse array of tests which assess a wide range of traits, it is pertinent to determine if a test is assessing the trait or theoretical construct it purports to. Therefore, one cannot simply inquire whether a test is valid, but rather "Valid for what?" Validity is very situation specific.[10] There are several types of validity:

Construct validity provides evidence to support a particular hypothesis or clinical theory. For example, Birch[11] postulated an orderly ontogenetic shift in sensory dominance. The shift would be from the proximal senses such as tactile to the teleoreceptor senses such as audition and vision. He observed that much of what is involved in the lack of readiness to read in grade 1 may be attributed to the fact that the final hierarchical shift to visual dominance had not taken place. Solan and Mozlin have shown that the time to complete the Six Figure Divided Formboard correlates with learning readiness in kindergarten[1] and with reading in grade 1.[12] Those children who are tactile and require a longer time to complete the task are more likely to be poorer readers at the end of grade 1, while those who are highly visual and have good spatial perception complete the task more rapidly and are more likely to be better readers at the end of grade 1. The correlations in the study support Birch's hypothesis. The test has construct validity.

When a second construct can also be identified by observing the child's cognitive style while assembling the Six Figure Divided Formboard, it suggests that concepts (constructs) may be interrelated. The impulsive child often uses a tactile approach which consumes more time to complete the task, while the reflective child who uses a visual approach to form the spatial match completes the task in less time. In general, it is probable that reflective children are more visual and are better readers than impulsive children who are more tactile. Investigating construct validity helps us to understand the trait(s) which a test measures and plan a treatment regimen which is more meaningful.

Content validity is applicable to optometric as well as school tests. For example, before using a non-motor test of visual perceptual skills, such as the TVPS, the optometrist should be concerned that all of the factors that would provide a comprehensive assessment of visual perception are included in the test battery. Further, the author of the test should indicate whether each item in a subtest (e.g., visual memory) correlates with the total subtest score. Since the test battery usually applies to a significant age range, do the items correlate with chronological age? In addition, the test manual should be reviewed to be certain that the test has been standardized and normed for the child's age. If not, the optometrist can not be sure whether the child has (or should have) the developmental framework to respond to the test.

Concurrent validity is present when two tests that measure similar traits correlate significantly with each other at one point in time. Concurrent validity is not judgmental. If one of the tests has preceded the other, and it has been considered the "standard," then it may also be considered the criterion. When a new test is introduced, the optometrist must ask: "What advantages does the new test offer with respect to standardization, norms and content?"

On several occasions, we have referred to the Six Figure Divided Form Board. It would not be reasonable to measure the concurrent validity between this test and reading in kindergarten since the child's reading skills are usually limited. It would, however, be valuable to know the relationship between the Six Figure Divided Form Board Test at the end of kindergarten and reading at the end of grade 1. This is a measure of *predictive validity*. Predictive validity is more accurate for groups than for individuals. From this information, perhaps we could predict the reading scores of a group of children at the end of grade 1 from the perception scores at the end of kindergarten. Solan and Mozlin showed that when *three* perceptual tests (tachistoscope, Six Figure Divided Form Board, and Auditory Visual Integration Test) were administered in kindergarten, 33% of the variations in reading vocabulary scores at the end of grade one could be accounted for by these three tests.[12] Although the predictive validity of the perceptual findings was significantly greater than that of the readiness test which had been used at the school, this information also told us that there were other factors which influenced the child's reading ability such as intelligence, motivation, educational opportunities and socio-economic status.

EPILOGUE

Readers who have come this far might well find themselves with a somewhat different clinical outlook than when they started this monograph. Some will be uncomfortable with the realization that a number of the clinical probes they've been using are not well standardized and/or offer inadequate yardsticks against which to compare patient performance. While they might continue using these tests, the results will be viewed more conservatively, and applied to diagnostics and patient management more cautiously. Still others will come away with a new appreciation that while no test is perfect, clinical care is enhanced by using probes that minimize ambiguity of the scores and maximize more precise interpretation of patient performance. Ideally, over time such concerns will generalize and result in a more sophisticated level of clinical thinking. The individual who has achieved this will appraise both existing and new tests, be they for visual perception or glaucoma, in a more critical manner. Questions regarding the characteristics of the sample of the population used to obtain normative data will be posed; the reliability of the test will be scrutinized; the clinician will be able to determine whether there is evidence that the test measures that which it purports. Further, the effectiveness of any treatment strategy will be evaluated not only from anecdotal evidence but also in terms of statistical significance. Performance or findings will be viewed not only in relation to the patient *per se,* but additionally in comparison to others of the same age, IQ and/or socio-economic status.

The attainment of this type of clinical thinking requires the application of virtually all the material discussed in this monograph to all aspects of daily patient care. The principles of Tests and Measurements apply not only to tests of visual perception, but also to procedures that evaluate the retina, accommodation, fusion, and virtually all clinical entities. We believe it is worth the time and effort that will be required. The optometrist will gain a new sense of certainty and confidence about his or her ability to make decisions, which is the outcome of all clinical encounters; and patient care will be enhanced, which is, after all, the prime responsibility of the clinician.

SELF ASSESSMENT

Part I

(Select best answer for each of 20 questions.)

1. Optometrists should be interested in learning more about Tests and Measurements (T&M) because

   a. school and other professional reports utilize the language of T&M and statistics to describe the patient's status.

   b. it is often necessary to appraise the clinical value of a new test for reliability and validity.

   c. it is important to know whether the treatment rendered to the patient has resulted in a significant improvement.

   d. all of the above are true.

2. Impressionistic testing has the advantage of providing

   a. more objective data.

   b. measures of separate specific traits.

   c. information of how a subject solves a problem.

   d. more reliable test results.

3. A test is an objective and standardized measure of a sample of behavior. By *standardized*, we mean

   a. all test questions should follow the same format.

   b. every examiner should conform to using exactly the same procedures and testing instruments when administering the test.

c. only standard scores are used in evaluating the test results.

d. the test is a valid predictor of a particular skill or behavior.

4. Norms are *not* characterized by which of the following?

a. may be within group or developmental.

b. provide direct information about the repeatability of a test.

c. are only meaningful when standardized procedures were used in testing.

d. the larger and more representative the sample, the smaller will be the sampling error.

5. The mean score of a group of 50 children tested

a. is not affected by extreme scores.

b. would be the same regardless of the number of subjects tested.

c. does not affect the standard deviation or z score.

d. is simply the average score for the group.

6. Which of the following is not accurate?

a. any raw score that is exactly equal to the mean has a z score of zero.

b. when normally distributed raw scores are converted to z scores, the shape of the curve remains the same.

c. the z score expresses the distance of an individual's raw score from the mean in terms of the standard deviation.

d. a z score of +1 represents a greater deviation from the mean than a z score of -1.

7. The mean, media, and mode all measure

    a. deviation.

    b. central tendency.

    c. frequency distribution.

    d. none of the above.

8. The percentile score is

    a. the percentage of items a subject answered correctly.

    b. the percentage of subjects that answer correctly.

    c. the proportion of a group getting a lower score.

    d. the probability of passing a test.

9 Which of the following is not true?

    a. z scores are readily convertible to percentiles.

    b. range is a rather crude measure of variability.

    c. mental age scores are important to know since IQ scores, such as the WISC-R, are determined by the ratio MA/CA = IQ.

    d. a child who is experiencing one year of retardation at age 5 is further behind than a child at age 10 with the same retardation.

10. Grade norms are useful because

    a. in any one subject learning is linear during the elementary school years.

b. it is easy to compare two subjects such as reading and arithmetic.

c. they provide exact grade levels of a child's performance.

d. in situations when supplementary instruction is provided, it is easier to explain the progress being made.

11. If testing 100 subjects results in 68% of the subjects having raw scores between 40 and 60, then

→ reliability is .8 then Var =80%

a. the variance is 100.   error Var =20%

b. 16% of the subjects should score below 35.

c. 70 represents a z score of +1.

d. a scaled score of 13 is equivalent to a raw score of 85.

12. In order for a test to have a high degree of reliability,

a. it must have standardized procedures.

b. it must have good norms.

c. individuals must maintain their relative ranks when the test is readministered.

d. all of the above.

13. If the reliability of a test (r_{tt}) is .85,

a. 15% of the total measurement variance is error variance.

b. 85% of the total measurement variance is error variance.

c. 15% of the total measurement variance is true variance.

d. the information to determine the error variance is insufficient.

14. Which of the following would probably lead to a decrease in the reliability of a test?

 a. increasing the homogeneity of the group tested.

 b. increasing the number of very difficult questions.

 c. decreasing the number of items in the test.

 d. all of the above.

15. The standard error of measurement (SEM) of a test with reliability of .89 and standard deviation of 15 is

 a. 13.4.

 b. 1.7.

 c. 5.

 d. 15.

16. The mean of a test is 50 and the standard deviation is 15. The standard error of measurement is 5. If an individual scores 37, the chances are 68 out of 100 that his true score falls within the range of

 a. 45 and 55.

 b. 22 and 52.

 c. 32 and 42.

 d. 35 and 65.

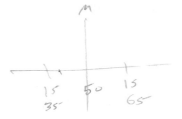

17. It is customary to retest an individual's skill after administering perceptual therapy. To be confident that the improvement is clinically significant, the difference in test scores should be at least

    a $\sqrt{2}$ SEM.

    b. 2 SEM.

    c. 1 SEM.

    d. 1 s.

18. Which of the following statements is true?

    a. A correlation of .50 is twice as strong as a correlation of .25.

    b. An increment in correlation from .45 to .65 is the same as an increment from .70 to .90.

    c. A correlation of r = +.50 represents the same degree of association as r = −.50.

    d. A correlation of r = .50 represents a probability of 50%.

19. The distinction between predictive and concurrent validity is

    a. mainly in the criterion used.

    b. the nature of the criterion data.

    c. the time that has elapsed between the test and the criterion.

    d. predictive relates to individuals while concurrent relates to groups.

20. Construct validity

    a. provides statistical evidence to support a particular hypothesis or clinical theory.

    b. is the least comprehensive type of validity.

    c. requires the use of blocks or copy forms to test.

    d. is principally determined by projective tests.

Part II

(Fill in correct responses for the following questions.)

1. For the following set of data:
10, 9, 8, 7, 6, 5, 4
Calculate standard deviation (s) and variance (V):
s = _____ V = _____

2. The mean and standard deviation for a test are 20 and 2. One hundred students took the test.

    a. What is the z score for a raw score of 24?

    b. What is the z score for a raw score of 19?

    c. Assuming that the test scores were normally distributed, what percentage of the scores would fall between the raw scores of 18 and 22?

    d. How many scores would fall between 18 and 22?

    e. What is the z score for a raw score of 20?

    f. What fraction of the students (approximately) scored greater than 22?

    g. On a test whose distribution is approximately normal with a mean of 50 and a standard deviation of 10, the results for three students were reported as follows:

Student A has a raw score of 65.

Student B has a percentile rank of 70.

Student C has a standard (z) score of 1.00.

Rank the order of the three students from high to low.

(A) ABC   (B) ACB   (C) BAC   (D) CAB

Part III

(Fill in correct responses for the following questions.)

1. What percent of cases fall between:

   a. −1 s and +1 s?   _____

   b. −2 s and +2 s?   _____

   c. −3 s and +3 s?   _____

2. What percent of cases fall above:

   a. −2 s?   _____

   b. −1 s?   _____

   c.   0 s?   _____

   d. +1 s?   _____

   e. +2 s?   _____

3. What percent of cases fall between the mean and:

   a. +2 s?   _____

   b. +3 s?   _____

   c. −1 s?   _____

   d. −2 s?   _____

NB: Work from normal curve and tables.

Answers to Self Assessment Questions

Part I

1 (d); 2 (c); 3 (b); 4 (b); 5 (d); 6 (d); 7 (b); 8 (c); 9 (c); 10 (d); 11 (a); 12 (d); 13 (a); 14 (d); 15 (c); 16 (c); 17 (b); 18 (c); 19 (c); 20 (a).

Part II

1. $s = 2$. $V = 4$.

2. a. 2.

    b. -.5

    c. 68%

    d. 68

    e. 0

    f. 1/6

3. ACB

Part III

1. a. 68.26

    b. 95.44

    c. 99.72

2. a. 97.71

    b. 84.12

    c. 50

    d. 15.86

    e. 2.27

3. a. 47.72

   b. 49.86

   c. 34.13

   d. 47.72

NB: You may wish to "round out" your answers.

REFERENCES

1. Solan HA, Mozlin R, Rumpf D. The relationship of perceptual- motor development to learning readiness in kindergarten: A multivariate analysis. J Learning Disabilities,1985;18(6):337- 344.

2. Solan HA, Mozlin R, Rumpf D. Selected perceptual norms and their relationship to reading in kindergarten and the primary grades. J Am Optom Assoc, 1985;56(6):458-466.

3. Anastasi A. Psychological testing, 6th ed. New York:Macmillan Publishing, 1988.

4. Hendrickson HH. Behavioral optometry approach to lens prescribing. Santa Ana, CA: Optom Exten Prog, 1980.

5. Nunnally JC. Introduction to statistics for psychology and education. New York: McGraw-Hill, 1975.

6. Guilford JP, Fruchter B. Fundamental statistics in psychology and education, 6th ed. New York: Mc-Graw-Hill, 1978.

7. Wechsler D. Wechsler Intelligence Scale for Children-Revised (WISC-R). San Antonio, TX: The Psychological Corp, 1974.

8. Piaget J. The origins of intelligence in children. New York: International University Press, 1966.

9. Suchoff IB. Cognitive development: Piaget's theory. Duncan, OK: Optom Extension Prog, Curriculum II, Ser.1, #4, 1978.

10. Brown FG. Principles of educational and psychological testing, 2nd ed. New York: Holt, Rinehart, Winston, 1976.

11. Birch HG. Dyslexia and the maturation of visual function. In J. Money (ed.): Reading Disability: Progress and research needs in dyslexia. Baltimore: Johns Hopkins Press, 1962;161-169.

12. Solan HA, Mozlin R. The correlations of perceptual-motor maturation to readiness and reading in kindergarten and the primary grades. J Am Optom Assoc, 1986;57(1):28-35.

APPENDIX

Sources of Testing Materials

1. Six Figure Divided Form Board
   Childcare
   1122 East 3rd Street
   Loveland, CO 80537

2. Grooved Peg Board Test
   Lafayette Instrument Company
   P.O. Box 5729, Sagamme Parkway
   Lafayette, IN 47901

3. Test of Visual Perceptual Skills
   Psychological and Educational Publications
   1477 Rollins Rd.
   Burlingame, CA 94010
   and/or
   VisionExtension
   2912 South Daimler Street, Suite 100
   Santa Ana, CA 92705-5811

4. Detroit Test of Learning Aptitude - 2
   Pro - Ed
   5341 Industrial Oaks Blvd.
   Austin, TX 7835-8898

5. Developmental Test of Visual Motor Integration-Revised (VMI)
Modern Curriculum Press
13900 Prospect Road
Cleveland, OH 44136

6. Tachistoscope
Instructional/Communications Technology (ICT)
10 Stepar Place
Huntington Station, NY

7. Auditory - Visual Integration Test
Optometric Extension Program Foundation
2912 South Daimler Street
Santa Ana, CA 92705

8. Wold Copying Test
Academic Therapy Publications
20 Commercial Blvd.
Novato, CA 94947

9. Gardner Reversal Frequency Tests
Creative Therapeutics
155 Country Rd.
Cresskill, NJ 07626

GLOSSARY OF FREQUENTLY USED TERMS

Correlation defines the type and degree of relationship between two variables, X and Y. As the correlation (between 0 and ±1) increases, the rank order of the scores of the subjects become increasingly similar. Correlational statistics are used to test hypotheses and to test whether the relationship between variables is statistically significant.

Mean is the arithmetical average of n measurements: the sum of n measurements divided by n. *All* measurements affect the value of the mean. Expressed as $\overline{X}$, it is usually accompanied by the standard deviation.

Median is the point below which one-half of the scores (50%) lie in a set of scores ranked in order from smallest to largest. Expressed as P_{50}.

Mode is the measurement that occurs most frequently. It is usually near or at the center of a distribution. May identify diagnostic entities that appear most frequently.

Normal Curve is a symmetrical bell-shaped distribution whose height (frequency, Y axis) is a function of the distance from the mid- point (mean/median) of the X axis.

Norms are scores that result from standardized testing of a representative sample of the population for which the test is designed. May be expressed as mean scores or a continuum based upon age or grade and expressed as raw scores, standard scores, age scores, grade equivalents, percentiles, and/or stanines.

Ordinal Scale represents members of a group that are ordered or ranked from most to least (or vv) with respect to a particular characteristic; e.g., locomotion, height, developmental stage.

Percentiles represent the percentage of individuals whose score falls below a given score. A percentile should not be confused with a percentage, which is a ratio. P_{84} is the 84th percentile.

Percent of Variance is measured by r^2 x 100 (r = .60; p<.0005; r^2 =.36; percent of variance = 36%). Provides information about the meaningfulness of the correlation. Using r = .60, it can be stated that 36% of the variations in the dependent variable (e.g., vocabulary, grade two) can be accounted for by variations in the independent variable (e.g., tachistoscopic exposure test).

Population is the data of all eligible people who have some observable characteristic; all of the members of a defined group: all of the members of an entering freshman class.

Range is the difference between the maximum and minimum scores. It is a good measure of how widely scores are dispersed, but it is not a robust statistic.

Reliability refers to the consistency or repeatability of a set of measurements obtained from a testing instrument. The reliability often varies with the nature of the population and the size of the sample.

Sample is a subset of measurements selected from the population that represents the relevant characteristics in the same proportion as they are included in the population.

Significance has a number of applications. In general, we are asking: "What is the probability that the obtained results could occur by chance alone?" Two specific applications follow.

1. **Correlation:** After computing correlation (r) from samples of two variables, we must determine the level of probability that the results are due to chance alone. That is, what is the probability that the true correlation is actually zero? For example, the correlation between visual processing with the tachistoscope and word recognition in grade one is highly significant (p<.0001), which means that the probability that the true correlation is zero is less than one chance in a thousand.

2. **Test-retest** is a procedure used frequently in vision therapy. After completing the therapy, what is the probability that the improvement in test score is statistically significant (p<.01)? Or, is the change in test results simply the product of errors of measurement?

Standard Error of Measurement (SEM) is, in effect, the standard error of the true score of a test. The obtained score falls between ±1 SEM of the true score 68% of the time. Since we know the obtained score, but not the true score, we often work in reverse, and hypothesize that the true score is within ±1 SEM of the obtained score. In practice, the SEM is used to interpret the accuracy of individual scores. *Good for pre/post testing to see*

Standard Deviation (S) is the average amount by which scores deviate from the mean in a normal distribution. *if improved*

$$s = \sqrt{\frac{\Sigma x^2}{N}}$$

Standard Scores in general relate to z scores, scaled scores, deviation IQs, and stanines.

1. z Score is the deviation of a raw score from the mean in terms of a standard deviation $[(RS - \overline{X})/s]$.

2. Scaled Score is a linear transformation of the z score that equals $10 + 3z$.

3. Deviation IQ is a linear transformation of z score that equals $100 + 15z$. It is sometimes called Perceptual Quotient.

4. Stanine is an abbreviation for standard and nine. Stanines are divided into nine subsets of scores. The mean is 5 and the standard deviation is 2. After arranging the obtained scores in descending order, then stanines can be formed. The scores are assigned in accordance with the following normal curve percentages:

Percentage	4	7	12	17	20	17	12	7	4
Stanine	1	2	3	4	5	6	7	8	9

Validity of a test concerns *what* the test measures and *how well* it does. The reader is cautioned to read the test manual carefully to learn how the validity of the test was established. "High" or "low" validity is not meaningful. There are a number of categories of validity.

1. **Concurrent Validity** is the correlation between the performance on a test and the criterion measure for the same sample of subjects. Often it is important to know the relationship between a single or a group of visual functional/perceptual tests and reading skills. Concurrent validity is an important concept for optometrists who treat children identified as learning-disabled.

2. **Predictive Validity** is similar to concurrent validity, except that the testing is carried out over a period of time. For example, perception tests performed at the beginning of grade one may be correlated with the criterion, reading comprehension skills two years later, at the end of grade 2.

3. **Construct Validity** is the extent to which a test measures a theoretical hypothesis, such as perceptual maturation from tactile to visual. For example, observing a child's strategy in completing the Six-Figure Divided form board reveals the level of perceptual-motor development.

4. **Content Validity** is an appraisal of whether the items in a test represent the behaviors that the examiner wishes to measure. Are the tasks appropriate and sufficient to satisfy the diagnostic objectives of the test? If the test battery is measuring non-motor visual perceptual skills in children, then the subtests should include all or most of the areas subsumed by visual perceptual skills such as discrimination, memory, form constancy, spatial relationships, sequential memory, figure- ground, and closure. The examiner cannot, however, generalize the results to predict whether or not the child will be able to conceptualize and/or copy a geometric form. If the tests are not carefully timed, then the norms do not provide information concerning perceptual speed.

INDEX

Split Half 31

Test-Retest 30

Sample

Behavior 5

Error 7-8, 9

Of Population 5, 7-8, 14, 17, 37, 62 (def)

Scores

Derived 14

Deviation 10-11, 13-16

Raw 6-7, 10-11, 15, 22

Scaled 2, 14, 19, 34, 64

Standard 1, 14, 19-20 (def), 24, 64

z 14-17, 19, 64

Self Assessment Test i, 47-55

Six Figure Divided Form Board 2, 16, 32, 38, 42-44, 59

Standard Deviation 1, 10-15, 17-19, 25, 28-29, 33-34, 37, 63

Standard Error of Measurement 30, 32 (def), 36, 63

Level of Confidence 33, 35-36

(SEM) Difference 34-35, 37

Stanine 64

Statistical Significance 38-39, 63

Tachistoscopic Exposure Test 4, 16, 44, 60

Test

(Def) 3

Standardized 4-5, 7